MULTIPLE SCLEROSIS DIET COOKBOOK

Friendly Recipes For Managing Symptoms, Boosting Energy, And Enhancing Wellness With Anti-Inflammatory, Gluten-Free, And Low-Sugar Options

DR ELIAN GRIFFIN

DISCLAIMER

The nutritional recommendations and recipes in this book are meant solely for informative reasons. They are not meant to replace the counsel, diagnosis, or care of a qualified medical expert. If you have any doubts about a medical condition or dietary requirements, you should always see your physician or another trained healthcare expert.

All reasonable efforts have been taken by the author and publisher to ensure that the information contained in this book is correct as of the date of publication. Recommendations may alter, though, as medical knowledge is always changing. When using any of the recipes or instructions found here, the user assumes all liability and assumes no risk, whether personal or otherwise. People who have certain dietary requirements or medical issues should speak with a healthcare provider for personalized guidance. The given recipes are only ideas; you may need to adjust them to suit your own nutritional needs, tastes, and tolerances.

When you use this book, you agree to release the publisher, the author, and their representatives from any liability for any claims, damages, liabilities, costs, or expenditures resulting from your use of the book.

TABLE OF CONTENTS

CHAPTER ONE 13

  MULTIPLE SCLEROSIS DIET INTRODUCTION 13

    WHAT IS THE DEFINITION OF MULTIPLE SCLEROSIS? 13

    HOW FOOD AFFECTS SYMPTOMS OF MULTIPLE SCLEROSIS.............14

    NUTRITION'S CRITICAL ROLE IN MS MANAGEMENT.................15

    SYNOPSIS OF THE MS DIET RECIPE BOOK.................17

    HOW TO MAKE THE MOST OF THIS BOOK 18

CHAPTER TWO 21

  FUNDAMENTALS OF DIET AND MULTIPLE SCLEROSIS.................21

    A SYNOPSIS OF MULTIPLE SCLEROSIS 21

    DIET AND MS: A CONNECTION.................22

    MS DIET TYPES 23

    ADVANTAGES OF ADHERING TO A PARTICULAR MS DIET PLAN 25

    ADVICE FOR ADAPTING DIETARY ADJUSTMENTS TO EVERYDAY 26

CHAPTER THREE 29

  GETTING THE MS DIET STARTED 29

    EVALUATING YOUR PRESENT DIET 29

    HOW TO GET READY FOR DIETARY ADJUSTMENTS.................30

    HAVING REASONABLE OBJECTIVES 31

    RECOGNIZING MS PATIENTS' NUTRITIONAL NEEDS.................32

    ESTABLISHING A FRIENDLY ENVIRONMENT FOR DIETARY 34

CHAPTER FOUR 35

  CRUCIAL ELEMENTS FOR MS ADMINISTRATION 35

    IMPORTANT ELEMENTS FOR MS PATIENTS 35

FOODS HIGH IN VITAL MINERALS AND VITAMINS 36

THE VALUE OF HYDRATION 37

SUPPLEMENTAL NUTRITION FOR MS PATIENTS 38

RECIPES FOR UPGRADING NUTRITION CONSUMPTION....................39

CHAPTER FIVE...41

ARRANGING WELL-BALANCED MEALS 41

FUNDAMENTALS OF A WELL-BALANCED MS DIET 41

EXAMPLE MEAL SCHEDULES FOR VARIOUS MS STAGES...................42

TIPS & TRICKS FOR MEAL PREPARATION 43

MODIFYING RECIPES TO MEET DIETARY REQUIREMENTS 44

A GUIDE TO GROCERY PURCHASING FOR MS-FRIENDLY FOODS 45

RECIPES FOR BREAKFAST..46

RECIPES FOR LUNCH 47

RECIPES FOR DINNER 49

CHAPTER SIX...51

COOKING METHODS AND ADVICE 51

RECIPES FOR HEALTHFUL COOKING FOR MS PATIENTS...................51

ADDING TASTE TO FOODS WITHOUT ENDANGERING HEALTH..........52

UTILIZING SPICES AND HERBS FOR EXTRA ADVANTAGES 53

KITCHEN UTENSILS TO HELP IN PREPARING MEALS.......................54

EASY AND QUICK RECIPES FOR A BUSY DAY...............................55

CHAPTER SEVEN 57

CONTROLLING SYMPTOMS WITH DIET 57

FOODS THAT COULD MAKE MS SYMPTOMS WORSE......................57

ADVICE ON HOW TO CONTROL FATIGUE WITH FOOD....................58

DIETARY TECHNIQUES THAT ENHANCE COGNITIVE PERFORMANCE .59

LOWERING INFLAMMATION WITH NUTRITION 60

RECIPES FOR MANAGING AND RELIEVING SYMPTOMS 61

CHAPTER EIGHT...63

EATING OUT AND INTERACTING WITH OTHERS........................63

GETTING AROUND IN DIETARY-RESTRICTED RESTAURANTS.............63

ADVICE ON EXPLAINING DIETARY REQUIREMENTS TO OTHERS 64

TAKING PART IN SOCIAL EVENTS AND FOLLOWING THE MS 65

SELECTING MS-FRIENDLY MENU ITEMS WHEN DINING OUT.............66

RECIPES FOR HOMEMADE RESTAURANT-STYLE DISHES 67

CHAPTER NINE 69

KID-AND FAMILY-FRIENDLY RECIPES 69

RECIPES THAT THE WHOLE FAMILY WILL LOVE 69

INCLUDING KIDS IN THE MEAL PREPARATION PROCESS...................70

MAINTAINING A HEALTHY DIET FOR THE ENTIRE FAMILY 71

CHANGES TO THE MS DIET FOR CHILDREN AND TEENS...................73

YUMMY & HEALTHFUL SNACKS FOR EVERY AGE 74

CHAPTER TEN 77

LIFESTYLE SUGGESTIONS FOR PEOPLE WITH MULTIPLE SCLEROSIS 77

THE FUNCTION OF EXERCISE IN MS MANAGEMENT..........................77

TECHNIQUES FOR STRESS MANAGEMENT 78

THE VALUE OF GETTING ENOUGH SLEEP 79

MANAGING MS DIET AND WORKLOAD...............................80

INCLUDING MINDFULNESS IN EVERYDAY ACTIVITIES 81

CHAPTER ELEVEN 83

FREQUENTLY ASKED QUESTIONS 83

HANDLING MS AND WEIGHT MANAGEMENT 83

HANDLING SENSITIVITIES AND FOOD ALLERGIES..............................84

MANAGING NUTRITIONAL OBSTACLES 85

MODIFYING THE MS DIET GRADUALLY 86

EXTRA RESOURCES FOR PEOPLE WITH MULTIPLE SCLEROSIS............87

ABOUT THE BOOK

The "Multiple Sclerosis Diet Cookbook" is an invaluable tool for anyone attempting to navigate the challenges of managing Multiple Sclerosis (MS) through dietary decisions.

It is important to recognize the significant influence that diet has on MS symptoms because nutrition is critical to improving general health and controlling individual MS symptoms. The book starts by giving a thorough description of MS, outlining its symptoms and how different dietary factors can affect the disease's course and outcome.

An important topic covered in this cookbook is the in-depth examination of various forms of MS diets, each designed to target particular requirements and symptoms that MS patients frequently encounter. By adhering to a structured MS diet plan, people may be able to reduce symptoms, increase energy, and improve their overall quality of life. Useful advice is offered on how to easily integrate these dietary adjustments into everyday routines, guaranteeing long-term benefits and sustainable adherence.

The focus of the cookbook is on essential nutrients that are critical for managing multiple sclerosis (MS). It lists important vitamins, minerals, and other nutrients that are important for immune system and neurological health, and provides helpful advice on how to incorporate these nutrients into daily meals through tasty and simple recipes. It also stresses the importance of staying hydrated and the role of nutritional supplements to supplement a diet.

The cookbook goes deeper into the concepts of creating well-balanced meals for various MS stages, providing readers with useful meal plans and strategies for effective meal preparation.

It also teaches readers how to cook in a way that maintains nutritional value while naturally enhancing flavors, so that dietary changes are not only health-conscious but also pleasurable and fulfilling.

It addresses particular symptoms, like fatigue and cognitive function, and offers diet strategies specifically designed to manage and alleviate symptoms; it also identifies foods that might aggravate symptoms and suggests substitutes that support reduced inflammation and general well-being. This comprehensive approach goes beyond preparing meals for oneself and includes eating out and socializing, offering helpful guidance on navigating restaurant menus and effectively communicating dietary needs.

Notably, the cookbook acknowledges the wider effects of multiple sclerosis on family dynamics, providing recipes that are inclusive of all family members and advice on how to involve kids in meal preparation. It also emphasizes the significance of preserving a nurturing atmosphere that promotes a healthy diet for people with MS as well as their loved ones.

Beyond dietary recommendations, the book delves into lifestyle factors that are essential for effectively managing multiple sclerosis (MS), such as regular exercise, stress reduction, getting enough sleep, and mindfulness practices. These factors work in tandem with dietary recommendations to promote a comprehensive wellness approach that supports both overall health and symptom management.

"Multiple Sclerosis Diet Cookbook" continues to be an all-inclusive manual enhanced with useful advice, recipes, and lifestyle suggestions meant to enable people with MS to make educated food decisions that improve their quality of life and overall health. It's a vital resource for anyone hoping to face their MS journey with courage and vigor.

CHAPTER ONE

MULTIPLE SCLEROSIS DIET INTRODUCTION

WHAT IS THE DEFINITION OF MULTIPLE SCLEROSIS?

A chronic autoimmune disease, multiple sclerosis (MS) affects the brain, spinal cord, and optic nerves; it develops when the immune system attacks the protective sheath that surrounds nerve fibers, misfiring and impairing nerve fiber communication and resulting in a variety of symptoms, such as fatigue, blurred vision, tingling or numbness, weakness in the muscles, and issues with balance and coordination.

The diagnosis of multiple sclerosis (MS) can be difficult because the disease's symptoms can vary greatly from person to person and can mimic those of other neurological conditions. Generally, the disease's symptoms can either worsen over time (progressive MS) or come and go (relapsing-remitting MS), and managing MS typically requires a multidisciplinary approach that includes physical therapy to improve mobility, medication to manage symptoms and slow the progression of the disease, and dietary changes to support overall health and well-being.

Comprehending multiple sclerosis (MS) entails identifying how the disease affects one's day-to-day functioning and navigating the difficulties associated with managing symptoms.

By addressing the disease's underlying mechanisms and implementing strategies to support neurological health, MS patients can improve their quality of life and more effectively manage its challenges.

HOW FOOD AFFECTS SYMPTOMS OF MULTIPLE SCLEROSIS

While there is no cure for multiple sclerosis (MS), diet can greatly impact the course of the disease and the severity of its symptoms. Certain foods have been shown to lower inflammation, boost the immune system, and improve brain health—all of which are advantageous for those who have MS.

In contrast, processed foods, sugars, and saturated fats can exacerbate MS symptoms by causing inflammation and impairing nerve cell protection. A diet high in fruits, vegetables, whole grains, and lean proteins, on the other hand, provides vital nutrients like vitamins, minerals, antioxidants, and omega-3 fatty acids.

Additionally, individuals with MS may find that certain dietary approaches, such as the Mediterranean diet or low-fat, plant-based diet, can help manage symptoms more effectively by reducing inflammation and improving overall health outcomes. Finally, maintaining a healthy weight through proper nutrition can reduce stress on the body and support overall mobility and energy levels.

NUTRITION'S CRITICAL ROLE IN MS MANAGEMENT

A well-balanced diet provides essential nutrients that support immune function, protect nerve cells, and promote brain health—all critical aspects of managing multiple sclerosis (MS). By emphasizing nutrient-dense foods and minimizing processed foods and sugars, individuals with MS can optimize their nutritional intake and enhance their overall well-being. Nutrition plays a pivotal role in managing MS by supporting overall health, reducing inflammation, and effectively managing symptoms.

A diet rich in a variety of fruits, vegetables, whole grains, lean proteins, and healthy fats provides the building blocks for cellular repair, energy production, and optimal brain function; this holistic approach to nutrition not only helps manage MS symptoms but also improves the quality of life and overall resilience. Proper nutrition not only supports physical health but can also positively impact mental and emotional health, which is crucial for individuals living with a chronic condition like MS.

Additionally, individualized nutrition plans that are customized to each person's needs and preferences can enable people with multiple sclerosis (MS) to actively participate in their health management. Consulting with healthcare providers, such as registered dietitians or nutritionists, can offer individualized advice and support in creating and adhering to a nutrition plan that satisfies particular dietary objectives and improves general health.

The MS Diet Cookbook is an all-inclusive tool created to assist people with multiple sclerosis (MS) in controlling their symptoms through diet. It provides a variety of tasty and nourishing recipes that are specially selected to enhance general health and well-being and cater to the particular dietary requirements of MS patients. All of the ingredients used in the recipes are well-known for their anti-inflammatory, neuroprotective, and immune-boosting qualities.

The MS Diet Cookbook is not just a compilation of recipes; it is also a guide to understanding the role of nutrition in managing MS and improving quality of life. With its wealth of information, recipes, and helpful tips on grocery shopping, meal planning, and kitchen organization, it is an invaluable resource for anyone interested in improving their quality of life and managing their MS symptoms.

People with MS can enjoy tasty and nourishing meals that support their health goals by incorporating recipes from the MS Diet Cookbook into their daily meal plans. Whether looking for ideas for breakfast, hearty soups, filling main dishes, or decadent desserts, the cookbook offers options that accommodate a variety of tastes and dietary preferences.

Each recipe is simple to follow, with ingredient lists and clear instructions that make meal preparation easier and empower people to take control of their nutritional intake.

HOW TO MAKE THE MOST OF THIS BOOK

To make the most of the MS Diet Cookbook, you should first become familiar with its contents and gain an understanding of how nutrition affects MS symptoms. Start by reading the introductory sections, which explain the fundamentals of the MS diet and the significance of particular nutrients in managing the disease. Next, make sure you have everything you need for meal planning and grocery shopping by going over the tips and advice provided.

When choosing recipes, take into account your nutritional objectives, dietary preferences, and any specific advice from your healthcare team. Look for recipes that include foods that are known to have anti-inflammatory and neuroprotective qualities, like leafy greens, berries, nuts, and lean proteins. Try experimenting with flavors and cuisines to make your meals fun and exciting.

Use the MS Diet Cookbook as a tool to learn about nutrition and discover new ways to support your health through delicious and nourishing meals. As you prepare meals from the cookbook, pay attention to how your body responds to different foods and adjust your diet accordingly. Keep track of your symptoms and overall well-being to identify any patterns or correlations between your diet and MS symptoms.

Discover new flavors, up your nutritional intake, and take charge of your health with mindful eating and nourishing cooking by incorporating the recipes and advice from the MS Diet Cookbook into your daily routine. This will help you manage your MS symptoms and improve your overall quality of life.

CHAPTER TWO

FUNDAMENTALS OF DIET AND MULTIPLE SCLEROSIS

A SYNOPSIS OF MULTIPLE SCLEROSIS

The complex autoimmune disease known as multiple sclerosis (MS) affects the brain and spinal cord, primarily the central nervous system. It arises when the immune system misattacks the protective sheath that surrounds nerve fibers, causing damage that impairs brain-to-body communication and causes a variety of symptoms, such as fatigue, blurred vision, tingling or numbness, weakness in the muscles, and issues with balance and coordination. The course of MS varies greatly from person to person, with some patients experiencing periods of relapse and remission and others having a disease that progresses steadily.

While there is currently no cure for MS, treatment aims to manage symptoms, slow down the disease's progression, and improve quality of life through medication, physical therapy, and lifestyle changes. Recognizing the unpredictable nature of MS and the significance of individualized treatment plans are important aspects of understanding the basics of the disease. Diagnostic tests, such as MRI scans and neurological exams, are used by medical professionals to assess the extent and progression of the disease.

Effective MS management necessitates a comprehensive strategy that takes into account lifestyle changes in addition to medicinal interventions. Since every person's experience with MS is different, tailored care is essential to optimizing results and effectively managing symptoms over an extended period.

DIET AND MS: A CONNECTION

Informed food choices can support medical treatments and potentially improve the quality of life for people with MS. The relationship between diet and MS centers around inflammation, gut health, and immune system function. Some diets aim to reduce inflammation in the body, which may help alleviate MS symptoms and support overall well-being. Research suggests that diet may play a role in managing MS symptoms and overall health.

A balanced diet high in fruits, vegetables, whole grains, lean proteins, and healthy fats can provide essential nutrients and support overall health; however, it is imperative that individuals with MS consult with healthcare professionals, such as registered dietitians or neurologists specializing in MS, to develop personalized dietary recommendations tailored to their individual needs and health goals. Certain dietary factors, such as omega-3 fatty acids found in fish, flaxseed, and walnuts, have been associated with anti-inflammatory effects that may be beneficial to people with MS.

MS DIET TYPES

The potential benefits of several diets, such as the Mediterranean diet, which emphasizes fruits, vegetables, whole grains, lean proteins, and healthy fats like olive oil, have been investigated for managing symptoms of multiple sclerosis and maintaining overall health. The diet is high in antioxidants and anti-inflammatory compounds, which may help reduce inflammation and support immune function.

Another well-liked strategy is the low-fat diet, which restricts the consumption of trans and saturated fats and emphasizes the consumption of healthy fats, like those found in nuts, seeds, and fatty fish. According to some research, lowering fat intake may help lower inflammation and possibly slow the progression of MS in certain patients.

Furthermore, the Wahls Protocol, created by Dr. Terry Wahls, promotes a diet high in fruits, vegetables, lean proteins, and healthy fats while avoiding processed foods, gluten, and dairy. The goal of this approach is to support mitochondrial function and supply vital nutrients, which may help MS patients feel less fatigued and have more energy.

It's crucial to remember that, even while these diets might have some advantages, there isn't a single diet that works for everyone when it comes to managing multiple sclerosis (MS). Instead, dietary suggestions should be tailored to each person's unique needs, preferences, and medical advice from healthcare providers.

ADVANTAGES OF ADHERING TO A PARTICULAR MS DIET PLAN

Adhering to a customized MS diet plan based on personal preferences and needs may provide multiple advantages for symptom management and general health support.

Antioxidant-rich diets, like the Mediterranean diet, can shield cells from oxidative stress and inflammation, which are common in MS.

A structured diet plan that meets nutritional needs can help some MS patients report improvements in fatigue, cognitive function, and mobility. Immune function, energy levels, and general well-being can all be supported by a well-balanced diet that includes essential nutrients, vitamins, and minerals.

In addition, following a nutritious diet can supplement medical interventions and lifestyle changes that medical professionals recommend, improving overall MS symptom management and quality of life. Nevertheless, patients with MS must collaborate closely with their healthcare team to track their progress, modify their diets as necessary, and guarantee the best possible outcomes for their health.

ADVICE FOR ADAPTING DIETARY ADJUSTMENTS TO EVERYDAY LIFE

With the right strategies and support, incorporating dietary changes into daily life can be a realistic and manageable process. First, educate yourself about nutrition and the various ways that different foods can affect your health and well-being, particularly when it comes to managing symptoms of multiple sclerosis (MS). You can also consider working with a registered dietitian who specializes in MS to create a customized diet plan that fits your preferences, lifestyle, and health goals.

Try reducing processed foods, sugars, and saturated fats and increasing whole grains, fruits, and lean proteins while reducing your intake of processed foods. Gradually adjust your diet by experimenting with different recipes and cooking methods to make eating healthy fun and long-lasting.

Stock your kitchen with wholesome foods, prepare meals ahead of time, and engage in mindful eating practiccs to create a supportive environment. Maintain regular hydration throughout the day by drinking lots of water; this can boost energy levels and general health.

Maintain contact with your medical team to track your progress, talk through any difficulties or worries, and modify your diet plan as necessary. By managing your nutrition and lifestyle proactively, you can better control your MS symptoms and enhance your quality of life.

CHAPTER THREE

EVALUATING YOUR PRESENT DIET

To manage Multiple Sclerosis (MS) with diet, you must first evaluate your current eating habits. To do this, keep a thorough food diary for a minimum of one week, noting down portion sizes, ingredients, and meal times. This will provide you with a clear picture of your dietary patterns and help you identify any unhealthy eating habits or potential triggers that may exacerbate MS symptoms. You should look for patterns such as high saturated fats, processed foods, or excessive sugar intake, as these are known to contribute to inflammation. Knowing your current diet is the first step in making decisions about the necessary modifications.

After that, review your food diary to identify areas that need attention. List foods that are good for controlling MS symptoms, like foods high in antioxidants, omega-3 fatty acids, and vitamins D and B12. Check the balance of macronutrients (carbs, proteins, and fats) in your diet to make sure you're getting enough of what you need. This assessment phase is important because it lays the groundwork for making specific changes that will improve your overall health and well-being. After carefully reviewing your current diet, you'll be better able to decide which foods to minimize or avoid.

HOW TO GET READY FOR DIETARY ADJUSTMENTS

To facilitate a seamless transition to a diet that supports MS management, there are a few practical steps you can take to prepare for dietary changes. First, familiarize yourself with the MS diet and seek advice from a healthcare provider or a registered dietitian who specializes in MS.

These professionals can offer individualized guidance based on your unique health needs and dietary preferences. Secondly, purge foods from your pantry and refrigerator that don't align with your new dietary goals and replace them with healthier options like fresh fruits and vegetables, lean proteins, and whole grains.

Set realistic goals for yourself regarding dietary changes, focusing on gradual adjustments rather than drastic overhauls. Prepare your meals and snacks in advance to avoid impulsive eating or reaching for convenient but unhealthy options. Invest in kitchen tools and appliances that facilitate meal preparation, such as a blender for smoothies or a steamer for vegetables. Stock up on essential pantry items like herbs, spices, and healthy cooking oils to enhance the flavor of your meals without relying on excessive salt or sugar.

HAVING REASONABLE OBJECTIVES

To effectively manage multiple sclerosis (MS), it is imperative that you set realistic goals. To start, identify specific objectives that are measurable and achievable, such as increasing your daily intake of fruits and vegetables or reducing your consumption of processed foods. You can then break down larger goals into smaller, manageable steps that you can incorporate into your daily routine, such as cooking at least three meals at home using fresh ingredients each week rather than relying on takeout or packaged foods. Progress should be tracked, and small victories should be celebrated along the way to maintain motivation and focus on your long-term dietary goals.

To successfully implement dietary changes that support your overall well-being, you'll need to set realistic goals that are in line with your lifestyle and health needs. Setting realistic goals will help you stay accountable and motivated. Seek support from family, friends, or online communities of people managing MS through diet. It's also important to be flexible and patient with yourself as you navigate dietary changes. Recognize that adjusting to a new way of eating takes time and may require experimentation to find what works best for you.

RECOGNIZING MS PATIENTS' NUTRITIONAL NEEDS

Identifying the dietary requirements unique to MS patients entails emphasizing foods that promote brain health, lower inflammation, and supply vital nutrients.

Antioxidant-rich foods, like fruits (especially berries), vegetables (especially leafy greens), nuts, and seeds, can help fight oxidative stress and inflammation linked to MS. Omega-3 fatty acids, which can be found in fatty fish like salmon, flaxseeds, and walnuts, are good for their anti-inflammatory qualities. Vitamin D deficiency is common among MS patients, so supplementation may be required.

Understanding these nutritional requirements and incorporating them into your diet can help support overall health and potentially manage MS symptoms more effectively. Protein sources such as lean meats, poultry, legumes, and dairy products (if tolerated) provide essential amino acids necessary for muscle maintenance and repair. Calcium-rich foods like dairy, fortified plant-based milk, and leafy greens support bone health, which is particularly important for MS patients at risk of osteoporosis. B vitamins, including B12 and folate, are essential for nerve function and can be found in fortified cereals, leafy greens, and animal products.

ESTABLISHING A FRIENDLY ENVIRONMENT FOR DIETARY ADJUSTMENTS

Establishing a supportive environment is essential to the successful implementation and maintenance of dietary modifications intended to manage multiple sclerosis. Begin by explaining your dietary objectives and requirements to your household members or close family to obtain their understanding and support. Inspire their involvement by having them help plan meals, shop for groceries, and prepare meals together. Make sure your kitchen is stocked with the necessary items and appliances to enable healthy cooking and meal preparation.

Seek out support from online forums, MS support groups, or local MS nutrition and management organizations. Exchange stories, recipes, and advice with others who are also navigating dietary modifications for MS. Think about consulting a registered dietitian or nutritionist with expertise in MS nutrition for professional advice.

CHAPTER FOUR

CRUCIAL ELEMENTS FOR MS ADMINISTRATION

IMPORTANT ELEMENTS FOR MS PATIENTS

Maintaining an adequate intake of key nutrients through a well-balanced diet is essential for managing multiple sclerosis (MS). Among these nutrients are omega-3 fatty acids, which are abundant in fatty fish such as salmon and flaxseeds. These fats have anti-inflammatory properties that may help reduce MS symptoms. Another important nutrient is vitamin D, which is important for immune function and bone health. Supplements, fortified dairy products, and sunlight exposure can help ensure adequate levels of vitamin D. Antioxidants like vitamins C and E are also beneficial; they can be found in citrus fruits, berries, nuts, and seeds.

Finally, maintaining a balanced intake of minerals like calcium and magnesium is essential for bone health and muscle function.

Green leafy vegetables, dairy products, nuts, and whole grains are excellent sources. By focusing on these nutrients through a variety of whole foods, MS patients can support their overall health and potentially manage symptoms more effectively. B vitamins, particularly B12, are important for MS patients as they support nerve health and energy production. Sources include meat, dairy, fortified cereals, and nutritional yeast.

FOODS HIGH IN VITAL MINERALS AND VITAMINS

For MS patients, a diet high in vital vitamins and minerals supports overall health and helps manage symptoms. Foods high in antioxidants, such as leafy greens, citrus fruits, and berries, offer a strong source of vitamins C and E, which protect against oxidative stress and can exacerbate MS symptoms.

Omega-3 fatty acids, which are important for reducing inflammation and supporting brain health, can be obtained from fatty fish, like salmon and trout. B vitamins can be found in nuts, seeds, and whole grains.

Dairy products and fortified cereals are sources of vitamin D, which is important for the immune system and bone health. Getting enough calcium and magnesium from foods like spinach, almonds, and yogurt is important for strong bones and muscles. MS patients can improve their overall nutritional intake and possibly even reduce some MS symptoms by expanding their food choices to include these nutrient-rich foods. MS patients can also benefit from balanced meals that include a variety of these foods.

THE VALUE OF HYDRATION

Drinking enough water throughout the day helps prevent dehydration, which can exacerbate fatigue and affect bladder function—two common concerns for those with MS. Choosing water as the primary beverage choice and consuming hydrating foods like fruits and vegetables supports optimal hydration levels. Hydration plays a critical role in overall health and can impact MS symptoms.

Maintaining cognitive function, energy levels, and temperature regulation are all important for MS patients.

Hydration is an important part of daily self-care for MS patients, as it can support their overall well-being and potentially help them manage their symptoms more effectively. MS patients can monitor their fluid intake and make adjustments based on their activity levels and the climate to ensure they stay adequately hydrated. Electrolyte-rich beverages, like diluted sports drinks or coconut water, can be beneficial after strenuous activity or during periods of heat to replenish minerals lost through sweat.

SUPPLEMENTAL NUTRITION FOR MS PATIENTS

Nutritional supplements can help manage MS symptoms in addition to a nutrient-rich diet. Vitamin D supplements are often advised, particularly for individuals with limited sun exposure, as they support immune function and bone health. Omega-3 supplements made from fish oil or flaxseed oil offer anti-inflammatory benefits that may help reduce inflammation related to MS. B-complex vitamins, such as B12 and folate, can support energy production and nerve health, which is often recommended for MS patients who are fatigued.

Integrating supplements into a comprehensive treatment plan, along with dietary adjustments and other lifestyle modifications, can help MS patients optimize their health and potentially alleviate some symptoms. Regular monitoring and adjustments based on healthcare provider guidance ensure safe and effective supplement use in managing MS. Antioxidant supplements, such as vitamins C and E, can be considered to help combat oxidative stress, which may contribute to MS progression. However, it's essential to consult with a healthcare provider before starting any new supplements.

RECIPES FOR UPGRADING NUTRITION CONSUMPTION

A well-balanced diet that supports overall health and symptom management can be maintained by MS patients by preparing nutrient-dense recipes. For breakfast, try a smoothie that contains leafy greens, berries, yogurt, and a scoop of flaxseed for omega-3s. For lunch, have a colorful salad with mixed greens, grilled salmon or tofu for protein, nuts or seeds for added crunch, and a vitamin C-rich citrus vinaigrette. For dinner, have a substantial dish of whole grain pasta with sautéed vegetables and a side dish of roasted sweet potatoes for an antioxidant and B vitamin boost.

Greek yogurt with berries and granola for extra calcium and magnesium can be a snack option. Energy-boosting snacks like trail mix with nuts, dried fruits, and dark chocolate offer a combination of antioxidants and healthy fats. Herbal teas or infused water with cucumber and mint can support hydration needs and complement meals. MS patients can enjoy tasty meals that improve their overall health and may even improve their quality of life by experimenting with different recipes that use nutrient-rich ingredients.

CHAPTER FIVE

ARRANGING WELL-BALANCED MEALS

FUNDAMENTALS OF A WELL-BALANCED MS DIET

Maintaining a consistent eating schedule is important to stabilize energy levels and manage symptoms. A balanced diet is essential for managing multiple sclerosis (MS). The principles center around making sure that meals are nutrient-rich, support overall health, and minimize inflammation. Pay particular attention to incorporating fresh fruits and vegetables, lean proteins, whole grains, and healthy fats into your daily meals. These foods provide essential vitamins, minerals, antioxidants, and omega-3 fatty acids that can help reduce inflammation and support nerve function.

A healthy diet is also important for MS patients. Drinking enough water maintains optimal body functions and promotes brain health. Processed foods high in sugar and unhealthy fats should be avoided because they can worsen MS symptoms by inflaming the body. Portion control is also important for controlling weight and making sure you get the right amount of nutrients without overloading your body.

EXAMPLE MEAL SCHEDULES FOR VARIOUS MS STAGES

Meal plans that are customized for each stage of MS can optimize nutrition and support overall wellness. In the early stages, emphasize foods high in nutrients that support the immune system and brain health. For example, a typical day might include baked salmon with quinoa and steamed vegetables for dinner, oatmeal with berries and nuts for breakfast, and yogurt with fruit or almonds for snacks.

More anti-inflammatory foods such as turmeric, ginger, and leafy greens can help reduce inflammation and support joint health. As MS worsens, meal plans may need to be adjusted to include things like smoothies with spinach, avocado, and berries for breakfast, lentil soup with whole grain bread for lunch, and a stir-fry with tofu and vegetables for dinner.

Fruit-based desserts, such as baked apples or yogurt with honey and nuts, can be used in place of desserts.

TIPS & TRICKS FOR MEAL PREPARATION

Meal prep makes the MS diet regimen easier to follow and guarantees that you always have wholesome meals available when you need them. To begin, plan your meals for the coming week, taking into account your schedule and dietary requirements. You can save time on busy days by batch-cooking staples like grains, proteins, and vegetables. Portion meals into containers so that you can easily grab and go, which helps you control portion sizes and discourages you from grabbing unhealthy snacks on the spur of the moment.

A range of healthy snacks, like fresh fruit, nuts, and yogurt, can help you curb cravings in between meals. By setting aside a few hours each week to prep meals, you can simplify your diet management and concentrate more on enjoying your daily activities. Experiment with different spices and herbs to enhance taste without relying on excessive salt or sugar.

Label and date your prepped meals to keep track of freshness and ensure food safety.

MODIFYING RECIPES TO MEET DIETARY REQUIREMENTS

For MS symptoms to be effectively managed, recipes must be modified to accommodate specific dietary needs. To begin, identify potential trigger foods and sensitivities (e.g., dairy or gluten) and adjust recipes accordingly. Replace ingredients with MS-friendly substitutes (e.g., almond milk instead of dairy milk, gluten-free flour instead of wheat flour). Try baking, grilling, or steaming to retain nutrients and flavors without adding excess fats or sugars.

Pay attention to the colors and textures you use in your meals to make sure you're getting a wide range of nutrients. For example, instead of using regular pasta, try zucchini noodles or spaghetti squash for a lighter, more vegetable-packed option. Use a lot of herbs and spices to add flavor and extra health benefits. When modifying recipes, pay attention to portion sizes and make sure each meal has enough protein, carbs, and healthy fats to support energy levels and general health.

A GUIDE TO GROCERY PURCHASING FOR MS-FRIENDLY FOODS

Choosing foods that support your overall health and nutritional needs when grocery shopping with MS entails starting with fresh produce, such as leafy greens, berries, citrus fruits, and cruciferous vegetables like broccoli and cauliflower. These foods are high in vitamins and antioxidants that can help lower inflammation and support immune function. Lean proteins, like those found in poultry, fish, beans, and tofu, provide essential amino acids without having too much-saturated fat.

Plan for meals and snacks and prioritize nutrient-dense foods to make the most of your grocery shopping experience while supporting your MS management goals. Whole grains, such as brown rice, quinoa, and oats, offer fiber and nutrients that support digestive health and stabilize blood sugar levels.

Healthy fats, such as those found in avocados, nuts, seeds, and olive oil, can help reduce inflammation and support brain health. Processed foods high in sugars, unhealthy fats, and artificial additives can exacerbate MS symptoms and contribute to overall inflammation.

RECIPES FOR BREAKFAST

Making wholesome and delectable breakfast options that promote overall health and energy levels is an important part of meal planning for people with Multiple Sclerosis (MS). A healthy breakfast can set the tone for the day, providing the necessary nutrients and energy to manage MS symptoms effectively.

You should also think about including foods high in antioxidants, vitamins, and minerals to support immune function and fight inflammation, which are common concerns for MS patients.

Start the day with a well-balanced breakfast consisting of whole grains, lean proteins, and healthy fats. Choose whole grain cereals or oats with fresh fruit and nuts to get fiber and important nutrients. Alternatively, go for a nutrient-dense smoothie made with spinach, berries, Greek yogurt, and flax seeds. These options are simple to make and adaptable to individual tastes and dietary requirements.

Try making homemade granola bars with dried fruits and seeds, or veggie omelets with avocado on whole-grain toast. These breakfast options provide long-lasting energy, which is important for controlling MS symptoms and enhancing general health. When nutrient-dense foods are prioritized and meal plans are well-balanced, people with MS can begin their day feeling good and supporting their health.

RECIPES FOR LUNCH

Planning well-rounded lunches for people with multiple sclerosis (MS) guarantees sustained energy levels and supports overall health. Lean proteins, whole grains, and plenty of vegetables are components of a well-rounded lunch that provide essential nutrients and support immune function.

If you have time, consider meal prepping to save time at lunchtime and guarantee nutrient-dense choices all week.

These lunch options are not only nutritious but also adaptable, meeting dietary preferences and nutritional needs. For example, try recipes like quinoa salad with grilled chicken and mixed greens, which offer a substantial dose of protein, fiber, and antioxidants. Alternatively, opt for whole grain wraps filled with hummus, fresh vegetables, and grilled tofu or lean turkey, which offers a satisfying and nutritious meal.

A balanced and comforting lunch can be made by trying homemade soups, like lentil or vegetable-based soups that are full of colorful vegetables and legumes, and serving them with a side of whole grain bread or crackers. By emphasizing nutrient-dense ingredients and well-balanced meal combinations, people with MS can enjoy lunches that support their health and well-being, encouraging sustained energy and symptom management.

For people with multiple sclerosis, a balanced dinner consists of nutrient-dense foods that support overall health and well-being. Lean proteins, whole grains, and vegetables are a good combination to provide essential nutrients and support immune function. Meal planning and delicious, nutrient-dense preparations make dinnertime easier and support optimal health.

Try baked salmon with quinoa and roasted vegetables for omega-3 fatty acids, protein, and fiber; or, for a satisfying and well-balanced dinner, try stir-frying lean beef or tofu with a variety of colorful vegetables over brown rice or whole grain pasta.

These dinner options are adaptable and can be tailored to meet specific dietary requirements and preferences.

Think about cooking in bulk so that you have leftovers for lunches or dinners later in the week. Homemade vegetable soups or stews made with beans and hearty vegetables are also great options for dinner, as they provide warmth and vital nutrients. People with MS can enjoy dinners that support their health and well-being by focusing on balanced meal planning and nutrient-dense ingredients, which can help with overall symptom management and vitality.

CHAPTER SIX

COOKING METHODS AND ADVICE

RECIPES FOR HEALTHFUL COOKING FOR MS PATIENTS

For people with Multiple Sclerosis (MS), cooking healthfully means utilizing techniques that maximize nutritional retention and minimize potential triggers. For example, instead of frying, try steaming, baking, or grilling to cut down on saturated fat intake, which can worsen symptoms. Steaming vegetables preserves their nutrients more effectively than boiling, preserving vital vitamins and minerals that are beneficial to overall health. Baking or grilling lean proteins, such as chicken or fish, helps maintain their nutritional integrity while adding flavor without excess fat.

To improve the absorption of nutrients, you may want to think about sautéing vegetables in heart-healthy oils such as avocado or olive oil. These oils offer vital omega-3 fatty acids, which are beneficial for MS patients because they have anti-inflammatory properties. You can also lock in flavors and textures by stir-frying with minimal oil, which keeps meals light and nutrient-dense. MS patients can benefit from tasty meals that support their overall health and wellness by implementing these cooking methods.

ADDING TASTE TO FOODS WITHOUT ENDANGERING HEALTH

A Multiple Sclerosis (MS) diet includes a creative use of herbs, spices, and natural seasonings to enhance flavor without using a lot of salt or sugar. Dried spices like turmeric, cumin, and ginger add depth to dishes while promoting immune health and reducing inflammation, which is beneficial for MS patients. Fresh herbs like basil, cilantro, and parsley add vibrant flavors and offer benefits like antioxidants and anti-inflammatory properties.

Homemade stocks infused with herbs like rosemary or thyme can add depth to soups and stews; citrus zest and juices can brighten flavors without adding extra salt, adding a refreshing twist to salads or marinades;

experimenting with different flavor combinations, such as sprinkling smoked paprika for a rich, smoky taste, can elevate meals while accommodating dietary restrictions.

UTILIZING SPICES AND HERBS FOR EXTRA ADVANTAGES

When used in cooking, herbs, and spices can offer MS patients health benefits beyond just improving flavor. Turmeric, for example, has strong anti-inflammatory properties due to its active compound curcumin, which may help reduce MS symptoms. Another anti-inflammatory spice is ginger, which can help with digestion and lessen nausea, which is a common issue for MS patients.

Incorporating these herbs and spices into daily meals not only diversifies flavors but also contributes to overall wellness. By harnessing the natural healing properties of herbs and spices, MS patients can enjoy meals that are both nourishing and delicious. Herbs like rosemary and sage offer antioxidant properties that support immune function and cognitive health, aspects that are important in managing MS.

KITCHEN UTENSILS TO HELP IN PREPARING MEALS

Having the proper kitchenware can make meal preparation easier for people with Multiple Sclerosis (MS). A good quality chef's knife and cutting board allow for the safe and effective chopping of fruits, vegetables, and proteins. Purchasing a food processor or blender can make tasks like pureeing soups or smoothies easier and guarantee that meals high in nutrients are easily absorbed.

Meal preparation becomes more manageable and enjoyable for MS patients when you optimize your kitchen setup with these tools. Non-stick cookware reduces the need for excessive oils or fats when cooking, promoting heart health and reducing inflammation—key considerations for MS patients. Adjustable measuring spoons and cups enable precise ingredient portions, supporting dietary adherence and nutritional balance.

When managing Multiple Sclerosis (MS), it's important to prepare quick and simple meals for busy days. For example, overnight oats made with rolled oats, yogurt, and fruits offer a nutrient-dense breakfast that requires little morning preparation, and stir-fries featuring lean proteins and a rainbow of colorful vegetables provide a balanced lunch or dinner option that can be made in less than 30 minutes.

Smoothies made with leafy greens, berries, and protein powder make for a filling snack or meal replacement on busy days. These recipes prioritize simplicity and nutrition, supporting the health and energy levels of MS patients amidst their daily activities. Salads with pre-washed greens, nuts, seeds, and a light vinaigrette dressing are quick to assemble and packed with essential nutrients.

CHAPTER SEVEN

FOODS THAT COULD MAKE MS SYMPTOMS WORSE

Some foods have the potential to aggravate symptoms in people with Multiple Sclerosis (MS). It is important to know what foods to avoid and how they can affect your condition. Foods high in saturated fats, like red meat and full-fat dairy products, have been linked to increased inflammation in the body, which can exacerbate MS symptoms.

Processed foods high in sugars and artificial additives can also aggravate fatigue levels and cause inflammation. Finally, some people with MS may be sensitive to gluten, which is present in wheat, barley, and rye.

The best way to control MS symptoms with diet is to emphasize whole, nutrient-dense foods, which include fruits, vegetables, lean proteins like chicken and fish, and healthy fats like those in nuts, seeds, and avocados.

Anti-inflammatory foods like leafy greens, berries, and fatty fish high in omega-3 fatty acids can also help reduce inflammation and support general health. People with MS can improve their quality of life and better manage their condition by avoiding or minimizing foods that may exacerbate symptoms.

ADVICE ON HOW TO CONTROL FATIGUE WITH FOOD

One major strategy for managing fatigue through diet is to maintain stable blood sugar levels throughout the day by eating small, frequent meals that include complex carbohydrates, lean proteins, and healthy fats. This helps prevent energy crashes and supports sustained energy levels. Fatigue is a common symptom of multiple sclerosis (MS) that can significantly impact daily life.

Another important strategy for overcoming fatigue is to stay hydrated. Throughout the day, make sure you drink enough water to avoid dehydration, which can make fatigue worse. Avoid caffeine and alcohol as these can cause sleep disturbances and increase fatigue;

instead, drink herbal teas or infused water to stay hydrated.

By including foods high in iron (lean meats, beans, and dark leafy greens), which can help fight iron-related fatigue, and foods high in vitamin B12 (fish, poultry, dairy products, and fortified cereals), which can support nerve function and energy production, people with MS can improve their overall quality of life and better manage their fatigue.

DIETARY TECHNIQUES THAT ENHANCE COGNITIVE PERFORMANCE

A diet high in antioxidants, found in colorful fruits and vegetables like berries, spinach, and bell peppers, can protect brain cells from oxidative stress and support cognitive function. Omega-3 fatty acids, found in fatty fish like salmon and trout, as well as in walnuts and flaxseeds, are also beneficial for brain health. People with MS may experience cognitive dysfunction, so it's important to adopt dietary strategies that support brain health and function.

Including whole grains, like quinoa and oats, as well as lean proteins and healthy fats in meals can help maintain steady energy levels and support brain function. Avoiding refined sugars and processed foods that can cause blood sugar spikes and crashes is important for cognitive health. Regular, balanced meals can support cognitive function by providing a steady supply of glucose to the brain.

Adopting these dietary strategies can help people with MS optimize their cognitive function and improve their overall well-being. Drinking water throughout the day and consuming hydrating foods like fruits and vegetables can support brain health. Even mild dehydration can impair concentration and memory.

LOWERING INFLAMMATION WITH NUTRITION

A diet high in antioxidants and phytonutrients can help reduce inflammation in the body and support overall health, as inflammation plays a major role in the progression of MS symptoms. A diet high in whole, plant-based foods, such as fruits, vegetables, legumes, and whole grains, can help reduce inflammation in the body.

Limiting the intake of foods high in processed foods, fried foods, and sugary snacks and beverages can help lower inflammation levels in the body. On the other hand, incorporating foods rich in omega-3 fatty acids, such as walnuts, flaxseeds, and fatty fish (salmon, mackerel, sardines), can help reduce inflammation and support immune function.

Incorporating anti-inflammatory herbs and spices such as turmeric, ginger, and garlic into meals can improve flavor and health benefits. Moreover, drinking lots of water throughout the day helps the body flush out toxins and reduce inflammation.

RECIPES FOR MANAGING AND RELIEVING SYMPTOMS

Making wholesome, tasty meals can be a big help in controlling MS symptoms. Anti-inflammatory ingredients and general health support are key components of recipes that help MS sufferers feel their best. For breakfast, try a smoothie made with spinach, berries, almond milk, and a scoop of chia seeds; it's packed with fiber, antioxidants, and omega-3 fatty acids that boost energy and reduce inflammation.

Protein, fiber, and healthy fats that support digestive health and satiety can be found in a quinoa salad with mixed vegetables, chickpeas, and a lemon-tahini dressing for lunch. For dinner, try grilled salmon with a side of roasted sweet potatoes and steamed broccoli, which provides omega-3 fatty acids, complex carbohydrates, and vitamins that support brain health and reduce inflammation.

Making nutrient-dense meals and snacks that support overall health can help people with MS manage their symptoms and improve their quality of life. Snacks like Greek yogurt with berries and a sprinkle of nuts can provide protein, probiotics, and antioxidants. Throughout the day, herbal teas and infused water can serve as hydrating and soothing beverage options.

CHAPTER EIGHT

EATING OUT AND INTERACTING WITH OTHERS

GETTING AROUND IN DIETARY-RESTRICTED RESTAURANTS

Navigating restaurants with dietary restrictions can initially seem daunting, but with a bit of preparation, it becomes manageable. Begin by researching restaurants in advance to find ones that offer options suitable for the MS diet. Many establishments now provide online menus or dietary information, which can be invaluable in planning your meal. When dining out, don't hesitate to call ahead and inquire about accommodations for special dietary needs. When you arrive, communicate clearly with your server about your requirements. Politely explain your dietary restrictions, emphasizing the importance of avoiding certain ingredients. Flexibility is key; sometimes, menu items can be customized to meet your needs. For example, asking for sauces or dressings on the side allows you to control portions and ingredients.

Remember to express appreciation for any accommodations made by the restaurant staff. Lastly, if the restaurant can't accommodate your needs adequately, don't hesitate to suggest another option or politely decline and choose another venue where your needs can be met.

ADVICE ON EXPLAINING DIETARY REQUIREMENTS TO OTHERS

Communicating your dietary needs to others effectively is crucial in social situations. Start by educating close friends and family about your MS diet and why it's important to adhere to it. Simple explanations can help others understand your needs better. When attending social gatherings or events where food is served, consider informing the host or organizer in advance about your dietary restrictions. This allows them to plan accordingly or inform you of the menu choices available. Politely remind your host about your needs, ensuring they are aware of any specific ingredients to avoid.

At larger gatherings, such as weddings or parties, discreetly ask the serving staff or caterers about ingredients in dishes before selecting what to eat. If necessary, be prepared to bring a small snack or dish that aligns with your dietary requirements to ensure you have something safe to eat. Above all, remain courteous and appreciative of any efforts made to accommodate your dietary restrictions, fostering positive interactions with others while maintaining your health.

TAKING PART IN SOCIAL EVENTS AND FOLLOWING THE MS DIET

With a few strategies, it is possible to enjoy social gatherings without giving in to the urge to overindulge in foods that may not be in line with your dietary restrictions. First, concentrate on the social aspect of the event rather than just the food. Second, engage in conversations and activities to divert your attention from any food-related worries. Third, if you can, eat a balanced meal or snack before arriving to curb hunger and lessen the temptation to eat foods that may not be in line with your dietary needs. Fourth, when choosing from the options available, give priority to whole foods like lean proteins, fruits, and vegetables, which are generally safer choices for the MS diet. Finally, think about bringing a dish or snack that you can enjoy and share with others, so you can make sure to

SELECTING MS-FRIENDLY MENU ITEMS WHEN DINING OUT

Choosing MS-friendly options when eating out requires a strategic approach to menu selection. Begin by scanning the menu for dishes that emphasize lean proteins, such as grilled chicken or fish, which provide essential nutrients without excessive saturated fats. Opt for dishes that incorporate plenty of fresh vegetables or salads, which are rich in vitamins and antioxidants beneficial for MS management. Avoid dishes that are heavily processed, fried, or high in sugars, as these can exacerbate inflammation and fatigue associated with MS. When in doubt, don't hesitate to ask your server about ingredient specifics or preparation methods to ensure they align with your dietary needs. Consider requesting substitutions or modifications, such as replacing fries with a side salad or asking for sauces on the side to control portions and ingredients. Staying hydrated is also essential; opt for water or herbal teas rather than sugary beverages to support overall health. By making informed choices and advocating for your dietary preferences, you can enjoy dining out while supporting your MS management goals.

RECIPES FOR HOMEMADE RESTAURANT-STYLE DISHES

Creating restaurant-inspired meals at home allows you to enjoy flavorful dishes while maintaining control over ingredients that suit your MS diet. Start by selecting recipes that emphasize whole, unprocessed ingredients such as fresh vegetables, lean proteins, and whole grains. Look for recipes that use herbs and spices to enhance flavor without relying on excessive salt or sugar. For example, try preparing grilled chicken with a side of quinoa and roasted vegetables seasoned with herbs like rosemary and thyme.

Experiment with different cuisines that align with MS-friendly dietary principles, such as Mediterranean or Japanese cuisine, which often feature ingredients beneficial for managing inflammation. Utilize online resources or cookbooks focused on health-conscious cooking to discover new recipes and cooking techniques that suit your preferences. Incorporate meal planning into your routine to ensure you have ingredients on hand for preparing nutritious meals at home. By exploring new recipes and flavors, you can enjoy satisfying meals that support your MS management goals while fostering culinary creativity in your kitchen.

CHAPTER NINE

KID-AND FAMILY-FRIENDLY RECIPES

RECIPES THAT THE WHOLE FAMILY WILL LOVE

Developing recipes that satisfy every member of the family can be difficult, but it's also gratifying. The secret is to strike a balance between nutrition and personal preferences. To begin, select ingredients that are easily modified to suit individual tastes.

For instance, stir-fries, tacos, and pasta dishes can be made to order. Adding a range of colors and textures to meals guarantees a varied intake of nutrients.

To accommodate dietary preferences, think about including family members in meal planning. This approach promotes inclusivity and encourages everyone to try new foods. When preparing meals, concentrate on incorporating whole grains, lean proteins, and lots of fruits and vegetables. For example, a family meal can be created around a build-your-own salad or taco night, which encourages autonomy and fun at the dinner table.

Play around with different cooking techniques and seasonings to keep meals interesting and nutritious. Roasting veggies or adding herbs and spices to enhance flavors can make dishes more enticing to kids as well as adults. By providing a variety of options and enticing everyone to help prepare meals, you foster a family environment where eating healthily becomes a fun and shared activity.

INCLUDING KIDS IN THE MEAL PREPARATION PROCESS

Assigning age-appropriate tasks like washing vegetables, stirring ingredients, or setting the table can be a great way to involve kids in meal preparation and teach them about nutrition and culinary skills. It also helps kids feel included and builds their confidence in the kitchen. You can also consider meal planning with your kids and letting them select ingredients or recipes they find interesting.

Make the most of meal preparation time to teach kids about the importance of a well-balanced diet. Talk about the different food groups and motivate them to make healthy choices when they cook. For instance, demonstrate to them how to put together a balanced plate that includes whole grains, vegetables, and proteins. Easy recipes like fruit kebabs or homemade smoothies can be enjoyable to make and a great way to teach kids about nutrition.

Emphasize safety in the kitchen and teach them proper techniques for handling utensils and appliances. By involving children in meal preparation from an early age, you instill healthy eating habits and create enduring memories as a family. Cooking can be a playful and educational experience that begins with exploring different cuisines or trying new ingredients together.

MAINTAINING A HEALTHY DIET FOR THE ENTIRE FAMILY

Consider using a balanced plate approach, where half of the plate is made up of vegetables or fruits, a quarter is made up of lean protein, and a quarter is made up of whole grains. Mindful meal planning and an understanding of each family member's dietary needs are the first steps toward balancing nutrition for the whole family. Begin by making a weekly meal plan that includes a variety of nutrient-dense foods. Aim to incorporate lean proteins, whole grains, fruits, and vegetables into every meal.

When organizing meals, consider personal tastes and dietary requirements. For example, if a family member needs to follow a gluten-free diet, consider brown rice or quinoa as a replacement for products made with wheat. You can also include healthy fats like nuts or avocados to supply important nutrients and encourage fullness.

Promote hydration by making water the main beverage option and limiting sugar-filled drinks. Fruits, yogurt, or whole-grain crackers can be used as snacks to fuel up in between meals. Pay attention to portion sizes and steer clear of highly processed foods that are high in sodium and added sugars. By emphasizing whole, nutrient-dense foods, you make sure that every member of the family gets the essential nutrients they require for general health and well-being.

It is important to take into account the nutritional needs and preferences of children and teenagers when modifying the MS diet. To start, speak with a healthcare provider or dietitian to develop a customized plan that addresses specific dietary issues related to MS. Stress the value of sustaining a balanced diet high in fruits, vegetables, lean proteins, and whole grains to support general health.

Families should adjust their meals to include MS-friendly foods, such as foods high in omega-3 fatty acids, antioxidants, and vitamins. Fish, such as salmon or trout, is high in omega-3s; try mixing colorful fruits and vegetables into smoothies, stir-fries, or salads to make sure kids get a variety of nutrients.

Provide MS-friendly snacks like nuts, seeds, or yogurt with fresh fruit to promote energy and satiety throughout the day. By creating a supportive environment and involving them in meal planning, you empower children and teens to make healthy choices that support their well-being while managing MS symptoms. Encourage open communication with children and teens about their dietary preferences and any challenges they may face.

YUMMY & HEALTHFUL SNACKS FOR EVERY AGE

It can be fun and helpful to find nutrient-dense, kid-friendly snacks that will keep them full throughout the day. To start, provide a range of options, like fresh fruit, veggies with hummus, or homemade trail mix, which is not only nutrient-dense but also portable and easy to make for people who lead busy lives.

Provide accessible snack stations in the pantry or kitchen, where everyone can get healthy options such as low-fat cheese sticks, whole-grain crackers, or chopped vegetables. Let kids put together their snacks by giving them a variety of ingredients to choose from, which will help them become independent and develop good eating habits.

Incorporate fun and healthy snacks into everyday routines by experimenting with creative snack ideas such as fruit skewers, yogurt parfaits, or whole-grain muffins with added fruits or vegetables. These snacks can be made ahead of time and frozen for easy grab-and-go options. Steer clear of sugary snacks and use natural sweeteners like honey or maple syrup instead of artificial ones.

CHAPTER TEN

LIFESTYLE SUGGESTIONS FOR PEOPLE WITH MULTIPLE SCLEROSIS

THE FUNCTION OF EXERCISE IN MS MANAGEMENT

To effectively manage the challenges posed by multiple sclerosis (MS), exercise is essential. Regular physical activity has been shown to improve endurance, strength, and flexibility. Aerobic exercises, such as walking, swimming, or cycling, can enhance cardiovascular fitness and improve mood by releasing endorphins, which are naturally occurring mood enhancers. Strength training exercises, such as lifting weights or using resistance bands, can help maintain muscle strength and prevent muscle atrophy, which is common in MS patients.

Exercise should be approached in a balanced manner, alternating between aerobic, strength training, and flexibility exercises to achieve comprehensive health benefits.

Individuals with MS should customize their exercise regimen to their abilities and limitations. Beginning slowly and gradually increasing intensity can help prevent fatigue and exacerbation of symptoms. Additionally, incorporating exercises that improve balance, such as yoga or tai chi, can help reduce the risk of falls and improve overall coordination.

TECHNIQUES FOR STRESS MANAGEMENT

Effective stress management techniques can include mindfulness meditation, deep breathing exercises, and progressive muscle relaxation. Mindfulness meditation involves focusing on the present moment without judgment, which can help reduce stress and promote relaxation. Deep breathing exercises, such as diaphragmatic breathing or belly breathing, can activate the body's relaxation response and calm the mind. Managing stress is crucial for people with MS, as it can exacerbate symptoms and impact overall well-being.

Engaging in enjoyable activities, like hobbies or spending time with loved ones, can also serve as effective stress relievers. Prioritizing self-care and recognizing when they need to take breaks or seek support from healthcare professionals or support groups are important for individuals with MS. By incorporating these stress management techniques into daily life, individuals with MS can improve their overall well-being and quality of life. Progressive muscle relaxation is a technique that involves tensing and then relaxing different muscle groups.

THE VALUE OF GETTING ENOUGH SLEEP

Sleep disturbances are common in MS due to factors like pain, muscle spasms, and bladder issues. Establishing a regular sleep schedule and creating a relaxing bedtime routine can help improve sleep quality. Avoiding stimulants like caffeine and nicotine close to bedtime and creating a comfortable sleep environment, such as using blackout curtains or white noise machines, can promote better sleep hygiene. Getting enough sleep is important for people with MS because it supports overall health, cognitive function, and symptom management.

Before going to bed, the body can be signaled to wind down by doing gentle stretches or reading. Healthcare professionals can help address any underlying issues that may be causing sleep disturbances, such as pain or anxiety. MS patients can improve their energy levels, mood, and overall quality of life by prioritizing sleep and putting strategies to improve sleep quality into practice.

MANAGING MS DIET AND WORKLOAD

Planning meals and incorporating nutrient-dense foods, such as fruits, vegetables, whole grains, and lean proteins, can provide essential vitamins and minerals to support immune function and reduce inflammation. Avoiding processed foods high in sugars and saturated fats can help maintain stable blood sugar levels and prevent energy crashes. For people with MS, juggling work obligations with a healthy diet can be difficult, but it's crucial for managing symptoms and promoting overall well-being.

It can be beneficial to find quick and healthy meal options, like batch cooking or prepping meals, to save time and energy during hectic workdays. It's also important to stay hydrated, as drinking too much alcohol can worsen MS symptoms. Finally, under the supervision of medical professionals, adding dietary supplements, like omega-3 fatty acids or vitamin D, can support overall health and complement a balanced diet.

INCLUDING MINDFULNESS IN EVERYDAY ACTIVITIES

Practicing mindfulness meditation, even for a short while each day, can cultivate a sense of calm and improve emotional resilience. Mindfulness involves paying attention to the present moment with openness and acceptance, which can help individuals manage symptoms and cope with the challenges of MS. Mindfulness, involves relaxation, reduction of stress, and enhancement of overall well-being.

An individual with multiple sclerosis (MS) should experiment with different mindfulness techniques until they find the one that works best for them. By incorporating mindfulness into everyday activities, such as eating mindfully or practicing mindful walking, individuals can improve their awareness and appreciation of the present moment. Additionally, engaging in joyful and relaxing activities, like spending time in nature or listening to music, can promote mindfulness and reduce stress levels.

CHAPTER ELEVEN

HANDLING MS AND WEIGHT MANAGEMENT

To effectively manage multiple sclerosis (MS), it is important to maintain a healthy weight. Many MS patients experience weight-related difficulties as a result of changes in appetite, side effects from medications, or mobility issues.

To address weight management, concentrate on a balanced diet that includes nutrient-dense foods while monitoring calorie intake. Include lean proteins, whole grains, fruits, and vegetables in your meals. Portion control is important, so think about using smaller plates to help manage portions visually.

Staying hydrated throughout the day to support overall health and digestion is crucial. Regularly monitoring weight and closely collaborating with healthcare providers can help adjust dietary and exercise plans as needed to achieve and maintain a healthy weight.

Even simple exercises like yoga or stretching can help maintain muscle tone and flexibility.

HANDLING SENSITIVITIES AND FOOD ALLERGIES

A registered dietitian or allergist can help you create a personalized MS diet plan that eliminates allergens while ensuring adequate nutrient intake. Managing food allergies and sensitivities while following an MS diet requires careful planning and awareness. Start by identifying any specific foods that trigger allergic reactions or sensitivities. Common allergens include gluten, dairy, nuts, and shellfish. Keep a food diary to track symptoms and identify patterns.

It is possible to maintain a varied and satisfying diet while effectively managing food allergies and sensitivities with careful planning and attention. Carefully read food labels and look for allergen information to avoid accidental exposure. Experiment with different ingredients and cooking methods to create allergen-free meals that are still enjoyable and nutritious.

Consider joining support groups or online communities to share experiences and recipes with others managing similar dietary restrictions.

MANAGING NUTRITIONAL OBSTACLES

Living with Multiple Sclerosis (MS) often involves navigating dietary setbacks, particularly during times of illness or fatigue. It's important to approach setbacks with patience and flexibility. If you experience a setback—for example, overindulging in unhealthy foods or skipping meals because of fatigue—don't be too hard on yourself. Instead, concentrate on gradually going back to your MS diet plan and prepare simple, nutrient-dense meals that are easy to digest.

Maintaining healthy snacks on hand, like nuts, fruits, or yogurt, can help manage cravings and sustain energy levels throughout the day. Staying hydrated can support digestion and general health. Changing meal timings or portion sizes based on your current energy levels can also help manage dietary setbacks effectively. Engaging in mindful eating can help you reconnect with hunger and fullness cues, which can help prevent future setbacks.

MODIFYING THE MS DIET GRADUALLY

Work closely with healthcare providers and a registered dietitian to monitor your nutritional needs and make necessary adjustments. As MS symptoms evolve, your dietary requirements may change. For example, if mobility becomes more limited, focus on nutrient-dense foods that require less preparation time. The MS diet may need to be adjusted over time to accommodate changing symptoms, treatment plans, and lifestyle factors.

To support overall health and manage MS symptoms, think about including anti-inflammatory foods like fatty fish, berries, and leafy greens in your diet. Try different recipes and cooking methods to make meals fun and interesting. Keep up with research updates and dietary guidelines for MS management to make educated diet decisions.

By being proactive and flexible, you can keep optimizing your MS diet for better symptom management and overall well-being.

EXTRA RESOURCES FOR PEOPLE WITH MULTIPLE SCLEROSIS

Joining support groups or going to educational workshops can also offer opportunities to connect with others facing similar challenges. Another way to get useful support and information for managing MS through diet is to look for credible websites, books, or patient organizations that specialize in MS nutrition and lifestyle management. These resources frequently offer helpful tips, meal plans, and recipes tailored to individuals living with MS.

Stay proactive in seeking out resources that empower you to make informed decisions about your health and well-being while living with MS. Online forums and social media groups can be valuable for sharing experiences and learning from others in the MS community.

Consider consulting with healthcare providers who specialize in MS care, such as neurologists, dietitians, or physical therapists, to access personalized advice and treatment options.